I0843556

Introduction: Understanding Post-COVID Stress Disorder

Hey there, brave souls! We've all been on quite a roller-coaster ride with the pandemic, haven't we? Now, as we step into this so-called 'new normal', there's another challenge that we need to address: Post-COVID Stress Disorder (PCSD). You might be thinking, "What now? Haven't we had enough?" Well, as tough as it is, we need to face it head-on because you, my friend, are a warrior, and warriors don't back down.

Post-COVID Stress Disorder is a condition that affects some people following their bout with COVID-19. It's much like PTSD (Post-Traumatic Stress Disorder), but in this case, the trauma is specifically related to the COVID-19 pandemic. Now, this doesn't just apply to those who've been infected; it also impacts people who've faced extreme stress, loss, or anxiety during this time. PCSD can show up as recurring nightmares, heightened anxiety, avoidance behavior, and a constant state of fear or dread.

"Know thy enemy" - it's an old saying but rings true here. Recognizing the signs of PCSD is the first step in battling it. Are you constantly on edge, thinking that you'll contract the virus, even when you're following all safety measures? Are you struggling with the fear of losing loved ones to the virus? Is the news about the pandemic triggering panic attacks? Are you avoiding social interactions entirely out of fear? If you answered 'yes' to any of these questions, you might be dealing with PCSD.

It's Not 'Just in Your Head'

First thing's first, your feelings are valid. Period. Don't let anyone tell you that it's 'just in your head' or 'you're overreacting.' The pandemic has been a significant event in our lives, and it's normal to feel overwhelmed. So, let's make a pact right now to ditch the self-judgment and be kind to ourselves.

Dealing with PCSD

Yes, PCSD is a challenge, but remember, you're amazing! Here are some steps to help you navigate through this:

- Seek Professional Help: Therapists and psychologists are armed with tools and strategies to help you manage and overcome PCSD. It's not weak to seek help; in fact, it's a sign of strength to recognize when you need it.
- Mindfulness and Meditation: The good ol' duo of mindfulness and meditation can work wonders in managing anxiety and stress. Just a few minutes a day can make a significant difference.
- Balanced Lifestyle: Regular exercise, a healthy diet, and adequate sleep – the golden trio of a balanced lifestyle – can help improve your mood and reduce anxiety.
- Connect with Loved Ones: Reach out to your friends and family, share your feelings, and draw strength from their support. Remember, it's okay to lean on others.

Understanding Post-COVID Stress Disorder is crucial as we navigate the aftermath of this pandemic. It's okay to feel anxious, scared, or overwhelmed. Remember, dear reader, there's no 'normal' way to react to a pandemic. It's uncharted territory for all of us. But by recognizing what we're dealing with, seeking help, and taking care of our mental health, we can emerge stronger.

The Science of Yoga and Stress Reduction

Hello, you gorgeous seekers of balance and inner peace! Are you ready to dive into the mystic ocean of yoga and swim to the scientific shores of stress reduction? Yoga, my friends, is more than just twisty-turny postures and balancing acts; it's a tool, an ally, a secret superpower we all have to defeat the relentless nemesis we call stress.

Yoga and the Brain: A Beautiful Tango

Let's get nerdy for a moment and talk about the brain. When we're stressed, our brain gets lit up like a Christmas tree with hormones like cortisol and adrenaline. While they're great when we need to outrun a saber-toothed tiger, in our daily lives, they can wreak havoc, leading to insomnia, depression, anxiety, and even physical illness.

Enter yoga, our brain's best dance partner. When we practice yoga, our brain releases 'feel-good' chemicals, including serotonin, GABA, and endorphins. These fantastic guys counteract the stress hormones and literally help to reshape the brain's structure and function, promoting calmness, focus, and a general sense of "I've-got-this" wellbeing.

And let's not forget about the mighty Hippocampus, a region of the brain associated with memory and emotional regulation. Studies have shown that regular yoga practice can increase the size of the Hippocampus. In other words, yoga can make your brain bigger and better!

Yoga and the Body: A Symphony of Calm

Now let's shimmy down to the body. Chronic stress tightens the muscles, speeds up the heart, and constricts the blood vessels. It's like a never-ending heavy metal concert inside you, and not in a fun way.

But, when we breathe deep in a yoga pose, we invite our body to switch from the 'fight or flight' response to the 'rest and digest' mode. Yoga stimulates the parasympathetic nervous system, which is like a calming lullaby for your body. It lowers your heart rate, eases your breath, and tells your muscles, "Hey, you can chill now."

Moreover, by increasing your physical strength and flexibility, yoga also builds resilience against the physical symptoms of stress. It's like you're simultaneously the conductor and the orchestra of your body, creating a symphony of calm.

Yoga and the Mind-Body Connection: A Harmonious Partnership

Yoga strengthens the mind-body connection, helping us to become more aware of our bodies and our mental states. This awareness, or mindfulness, is a super effective stress-buster. By bringing your attention to the present, yoga helps you break free from the cage of past regrets and future worries.

It's like giving yourself permission to stop, breathe, and just be. By noticing the quality of your breath, the alignment of your body in a pose, and the flow of thoughts in your mind, you can identify signs of stress and counteract them before they snowball.

So, there you have it, the amazing science of yoga and stress reduction. This isn't some airy-fairy concept; it's real, it's tangible, and it's ready to be tapped by you, right here, right now. So, roll out that mat, strike a pose, and let the calming magic of yoga wash over you. You, my friend, have got the power. The power to reduce stress, to nurture your well-being, and to harness your inner calm. So get out there, be bold, be brave, and let your yoga journey unfold!

Start Small, Dream Big

The beauty of yoga is its flexibility (pun intended!). There's no need to jump into a 90-minute advanced Vinyasa flow from the get-go. Start with just 10-15 minutes a day. Pick a time that works for you - early morning, during lunch break, or before bed. The important thing is consistency. Even a few minutes of daily practice can yield positive results.

Your Body is Your Temple

Your yoga practice isn't about nailing the perfect headstand or twisting into a pretzel. It's about respecting your body, its capabilities, and its limits. So listen to your body. Some days, you might feel energetic and ready for a dynamic flow. Other days, your body might crave restorative poses. There's no right or wrong here. Remember, you're not competing with anyone, not even yourself.

Breathe Easy

Breath is the cornerstone of yoga. Make sure to incorporate pranayama or breathwork into your practice. You'd be surprised how something as simple as focusing on your breath can drastically reduce stress levels. Try techniques like Anulom Vilom (alternate nostril breathing) or Ujjayi (victorious breath) to stimulate relaxation. We will learn more about this later.

Find Your Zen Space

Create a personal space for your yoga practice. It doesn't have to be an elaborate yoga studio. Just a quiet, clean space where you won't be disturbed. Add elements that uplift your spirits - it could be scented candles, soothing music, or even a picture of a serene landscape. This space will become your haven, your escape from the daily grind.

Don't Skip Savasana

Finally, never underestimate the power of Savasana, also known as the corpse pose. It might look like you're just lying there, but Savasana is where the magic happens. This pose helps your body absorb the benefits of your practice and transition back to a state of rest. It's the perfect finale to your yoga session, leaving you feeling calm, grounded, and rejuvenated.

Incorporating yoga into your daily routine might seem daunting at first, but once you take that leap, you'll wonder why you didn't start sooner. Remember, yoga isn't just about reducing stress; it's about celebrating yourself, your strength, your resilience, and your journey. So embrace yoga with an open heart and a spirited mind. Take it one breath at a time, one pose at a time. This is your journey, and you are the author of your own yoga story. Now, go ahead, unfold that mat, take a deep breath, and let your journey begin!

Breathe In, Bliss Out: Yoga for Relaxation and Mindfulness

It's time to set your stress aside, awaken your mindfulness, and get ready to unwind with the ancient wisdom of yoga. Yoga is your own personal retreat, a sanctuary where you can breathe in peace and breathe out tension. So, let's delve into the world of yoga for relaxation and mindfulness.

Relaxation and Yoga: Unraveling the Knots of Tension

Relaxation, it sounds so simple, yet it's something many of us struggle to achieve in our fast-paced, always-on world. The stress of juggling work, family, social commitments, and the occasional curveballs that life throws our way can leave us wound up tighter than a ball of yarn in a kitten's paws.

This is where yoga comes in, like a warm hug on a chilly day. It activates our parasympathetic nervous system, the body's natural relaxation response. This slows down our heart rate, lowers our blood pressure, and helps our body and mind find calm amidst the chaos.

Yogic practices like Yoga Nidra, also known as yogic sleep, guide you through various stages of consciousness. They take you on a journey from the external world to your innermost self, allowing you to relax deeply. Even a simple pose like Savasana, or Corpse Pose, can trigger deep relaxation, helping to soothe both body and mind.

Ready to dive into the soothing ocean of Yoga Nidra?

Grab your mat, get comfy, and prepare to unlock a whole new level of relaxation and awareness. In this chapter, I'll guide you through a step-by-step Yoga Nidra practice. Let's get started!

Step 1: Prepare Your Space

Find a quiet, comfortable space where you won't be disturbed. Lay down your yoga mat, place a bolster under your knees for support if you like, and have a blanket nearby in case you get cold. Dim the lights or close your eyes to help focus inward.

Step 2: Settle into Savasana

Lie down on your back in Savasana, also known as Corpse Pose. Allow your legs to spread slightly apart and your feet to relax to the sides. Rest your arms by your sides, palms facing upward. Make any adjustments to ensure you're comfortable. Remember, comfort is key in Yoga Nidra!

Step 3: Set Your Sankalpa

Sankalpa, or intention, is a vital part of Yoga Nidra. Think of a short positive statement or affirmation that resonates with you, such as "I am at peace" or "I am filled with joy." It should be phrased in the present tense, as if it's already happening. Repeat your Sankalpa mentally three times with conviction.

Step 4: Perform a Body Scan

Begin to bring your awareness to different parts of your body, starting from your toes and moving up to the crown of your head. As you mentally name each part of your body, imagine releasing tension from that area. Take your time with this stage; it's a crucial part of the relaxation process.

Step 5: Dive into Breath Awareness

Now, shift your focus to your breath. Observe each inhale and exhale without trying to change or control your breath. Feel the cool air entering your nostrils and the warm air leaving. Notice the gentle rise and fall of your chest and abdomen as you breathe.

Step 6: Embrace Opposite Sensations

Next, you'll explore opposite sensations or feelings, such as heaviness and lightness, heat and cold. Imagine your body feeling as heavy as a rock, then as light as a feather. Then imagine the heat of the summer sun enveloping your body, then the coolness of a gentle breeze. This stage helps to deepen your state of relaxation.

Step 7: Visualize

In this stage, you'll visualize various images, landscapes, or experiences, as guided by the Yoga Nidra script or recording you're using. This could range from a peaceful beach to a starlit sky. Engage all your senses in this visualization.

Step 8: Return to Your Sankalpa

As your Yoga Nidra practice nears its end, mentally repeat your Sankalpa three times again, just as you did in the beginning.

Step 9: Ease Back into Awareness

Finally, gradually bring your awareness back to your surroundings. Feel the ground beneath you, listen to the sounds around you, and slowly start to move your fingers and toes. Roll over to one side and gently push yourself up to a seated position.

Congratulations, you've completed a Yoga Nidra session! This profound practice can lead you to an oasis of tranquility and heightened awareness within. With regular practice, you'll likely notice increased inner peace, reduced stress, and improved sleep. So enjoy this journey of self-discovery, and remember, each time you practice Yoga Nidra, you're taking a step toward your own personal well-being and self-growth. Shine on, you beautiful beacon of tranquility!

Mindfulness and Yoga: Embracing the Here and Now

Mindfulness is a beautiful gift we can give ourselves – the gift of being present. It's about waking up to the magic of the ordinary moments that fill our days. Yoga serves as an invitation to mindfulness.

When you're in a yoga pose, you're tuned into the rhythm of your breath, the alignment of your body, the sensation in your muscles. Whether it's the stretch in your spine during a forward bend or the strength in your legs in a Warrior pose, yoga nudges you to be here and now.

Pranayama, the practice of breath control, is another tool to enhance mindfulness. Techniques such as Anulom Vilom (Alternate Nostril Breathing) or Ujjayi (Ocean Breath) anchor your mind to the present, reducing its tendency to wander into past regrets or future worries.

Merging Relaxation and Mindfulness with Yoga

By integrating relaxation and mindfulness, yoga provides a holistic approach to stress management. The key is to create a yoga routine that includes asanas (poses), pranayama (breathwork), and meditation for a balanced practice. You can choose poses that promote relaxation such as Child's Pose (Balasana), Seated Forward Bend (Paschimottanasana), and Legs-Up-The-Wall Pose (Viparita Karani).

While practicing these poses, maintain your focus on your breath and the sensations in your body. This merges relaxation and mindfulness, helping you to let go of stress and find tranquility.

Building a Daily Yoga Practice

Building a daily yoga practice is like planting a seed of calm and nurturing it each day. Start with a short, manageable routine and gradually expand it as your comfort and familiarity with the practice grows.

Morning practice can energize and set a positive tone for the day, while an evening practice can help you unwind and release the day's stress. Choose what suits your lifestyle and needs best.

Yoga for relaxation and mindfulness is a journey, not a destination. It's about learning to navigate life's ups and downs with grace, embracing each moment with mindfulness, and finding peace within yourself.

Every time you step onto your yoga mat, you take a step towards better stress management, deeper self-awareness, and improved well-being. So roll out your mat, take a deep breath, and get ready to relax and reconnect with the glorious being that you are. Remember, in the hustle and bustle of life, don't forget to pause, breathe, and just be.

The Companion of Mindfulness: Cultivating Present Moment Awareness in Post-COVID Recovery

Welcome, resilient warriors! As we continue to explore the transformative aspects of yoga, pranayama, and meditation in your post-COVID recovery, let's illuminate another invaluable tool: mindfulness. In its simplest form, mindfulness is the practice of cultivating awareness of the present moment, a potent resource in navigating your path to wellness.

Why Mindfulness Matters in Post-COVID Recovery

In the aftermath of illness, especially one as globally impactful as COVID-19, it's not uncommon to find yourself dealing with stress, anxiety, and a sense of uncertainty about the future. Here is where mindfulness can play a crucial role.

1. *Stress Reduction:* Regular mindfulness practice has been linked with reduced stress levels. It encourages a shift from automatic, often stress-induced reactions to thoughtful, calm responses.

2. *Enhancing Emotional Well-being:* By focusing on the present, mindfulness can help minimize ruminative thoughts about the past or worries about the future, fostering emotional well-being.

3. *Supports Physical Health:* Mindfulness can help improve sleep quality, enhance immune function, and even aid in pain management, making it beneficial for physical recovery.

Strategies for Cultivating Mindfulness During Recovery

Integrating mindfulness into your daily routine doesn't require drastic changes. Here are a few simple strategies to cultivate mindfulness:

1. *Mindful Breathing:* This involves focusing your attention on your breath, observing the sensation of inhaling and exhaling. This practice can be done anywhere, anytime, and serves as a straightforward way to return your focus to the present.

2. *Mindful Eating:* Pay attention to the tastes, textures, and smells of your food. Chew slowly, savoring each bite. This practice not only enhances the eating experience but also helps improve digestion.

3. *Mindful Walking:* As your strength allows, take short, gentle walks. As you walk, pay attention to the sensation of your feet making contact with the ground, the rhythm of your steps, and your breath.

4. *Body Scan Meditation:* This form of mindfulness practice involves focusing your attention gradually and intentionally on different parts of your body, from your toes to your head.

5. *Mindful Yoga:* As you practice yoga, focus on your bodily sensations as you move through each pose. Notice how your muscles and joints feel and coordinate your movements with your breath.

As you embrace mindfulness on your recovery journey, remember that it's not about achieving a particular state or feeling. Instead, it's about becoming an attentive observer of your present-moment experiences without judgment.

By weaving mindfulness into your yoga, pranayama, and meditation practices, you can enhance your overall recovery process. Every mindful breath, every attentive moment, and every present-focused practice becomes a step towards recovery, adding to your resilience and strength.

Embrace this journey with patience and self-compassion. Each mindful moment is a step towards healing, each breath a testament to your resilience.

The Yin and Yang: Balancing Effort and Ease in Yoga

Are you ready to uncover a profound aspect of yoga that bridges the physical and the mindful? As we further our journey into yoga for relaxation and mindfulness, let's talk about the delicate balance between effort and ease.

Effort and Ease in Yoga: An Ancient Wisdom

The concept of balancing effort (sthira) and ease (sukha) in yoga comes from the Yoga Sutras of Patanjali, one of the foundational texts of yoga philosophy. Sutra 2.46 states "Sthira-sukham asanam," which translates to "Posture (asana) should be stable (sthira) and comfortable (sukha)." This teaching suggests that every yoga pose should be a balance of effort and ease, engagement and relaxation.

Balancing Effort and Ease: The Practical Approach

In practical terms, effort in yoga might mean engaging your muscles in a pose, maintaining proper alignment, or holding a pose for multiple breaths. Ease, on the other hand, could be maintaining a calm and steady breath, softening tension in your face or jaw, or finding a sense of comfort within the challenge of the pose.

The Role of Mindfulness

Mindfulness is the secret ingredient in balancing effort and ease. It's about being aware of your body and your breath, noticing where you're straining, and where you can soften. It's also about recognizing when you're pushing yourself too hard and when you need to challenge yourself a bit more.

A Mindful Practice: Balancing Effort and Ease

Next time you unroll your yoga mat, bring your attention to the balance of effort and ease in your practice. Notice where in your body you feel effort and where you feel ease. Are there places where you can soften or engage more? How is your breath influencing your sense of effort and ease?

Through this practice, you're not just enhancing your physical yoga practice; you're cultivating a life skill. After all, life, much like yoga, is a balance of effort and ease. We need effort to grow and achieve, and we need ease to rest and rejuvenate.

Balancing effort and ease in yoga is a dance – a dance between strength and softness, challenge and comfort, doing and being. This dance is not just performed on your yoga mat but woven into the fabric of your daily life.

As you continue your yoga journey, remember to embrace this balance. Some days, you might lean more towards effort, and other days, towards ease. And that's perfectly okay. After all, you're not seeking perfection, but harmony – the harmony between effort and ease, between the body and the mind, between the self and the universe. So keep dancing, dear yogis, and let your dance be as unique and beautiful as you are!

Rock Your Breath: Pranayama Techniques for Taming Anxiety and Depression

Are you ready to rock your life, trade stress for calm, and tap into that powerful energy that's waiting to burst free? Well, strap in because we're going to dive deep into the world of Pranayama, the yoga practice of controlling the breath. And, you know what they say about Pranayama - it's like a free Wi-Fi connection to the Universe. With each breath you take, you connect to your inner self and the calming vibes of the cosmos.

Breathing isn't just about keeping you alive - it's about feeling alive. When you control your breath, you can control your life. Pranayama practices can help you tackle anxiety and depression, those sneaky devils that love to sabotage your day. So let's delve into some juicy techniques to kick anxiety and depression to the curb!

1. Anulom Vilom (Alternate Nostril Breathing)

Anulom Vilom is like a super smoothie for your brain. This practice helps balance the left and right hemispheres, promoting a sense of calm and reducing anxiety. Here's how to do it:

- Sit comfortably, back straight, and shoulders relaxed. (Picture yourself as the queen or king of your own castle.)

- Close your right nostril with your right thumb and inhale slowly through your left nostril.

- Now, close your left nostril with your right ring finger, and exhale slowly through your right nostril.

- Inhale through your right nostril, close it, and then exhale through your left nostril.

- Repeat this cycle for about five minutes, and imagine your worries leaving with each exhale.

2. Ujjayi Pranayama (Victorious Breath)

Think of Ujjayi Pranayama as your personal superhero. This powerful practice can help lift your mood and take on depression.

- Start by inhaling deeply through your nose.

- Then, with your mouth closed, exhale through your nose while constricting the back of your throat, producing a soft ocean-like sound.

- Imagine yourself victorious over your fears and sadness with each breath.

- Practice this for five to ten minutes daily.

3. Bhramari Pranayama (Bee Breath)

Bhramari Pranayama is your private sound bath, and it's all about vibrating higher. The resonating hum in this technique soothes your mind, eradicating anxiety and depression.

- Close your eyes and take a deep breath in.

- As you breathe out, gently press your ears, humming like a bee.

- Repeat this for a few rounds, and feel the vibrations soothing your mind and uplifting your spirits.

Pranayama is a yoga superstar that lets you tap into your internal energy, flipping the switch from anxiety and depression to calm and happiness. Remember, gorgeous, the energy you create within you is the life you create around you. So, fill your lungs, clear your mind, and let that amazing energy flow.

And don't forget to take it slow and gentle. Pranayama is not a race, but a beautiful dance with your breath. Don't be hard on yourself if you don't get it right away. Be patient, breathe, and allow the magic to happen.

So, get out there and rock your breath.

Flowing with Mindfulness: Exploring Mindful Yoga Sequences

Hey there, mindful mavens! Ready to infuse your yoga flows with an extra dash of mindfulness? You're in for a treat! In this chapter, we'll explore some mindful yoga sequences that unite body, breath, and mind. So, unroll your mat, get comfortable, and let's dive in.

Yoga Sequence for Morning Mindfulness

Starting your day with mindfulness sets the tone for a calm, focused day. Here's a simple sequence to awaken your body and mind.

1. Begin in Mountain Pose (Tadasana): Stand tall, feel your feet grounding into the earth, and take a few deep breaths.

2. Flow into Sun Salutations (Surya Namaskar): This series of poses warms up the body and focuses the mind. As you flow through each pose, coordinate your movements with your breath.

3. Practice Tree Pose (Vrksasana): This balancing pose enhances focus and promotes a sense of calm.

4. End with a brief seated meditation: Sit comfortably, observe your breath, and set an intention for your day.

Mindful Yoga Sequence for Mid-Day Reset

Feeling a mid-day slump? Try this sequence to refresh your mind and body.

1. Start in Seated Spinal Twist (Ardha Matsyendrasana): This pose helps to relieve tension in the back and shoulders, areas where we often hold stress.

2. Move into Cat-Cow Pose (Marjaiasana-Bitilasana): This pair of poses helps to release tension in the spine and neck, while connecting your movement and breath.

3. Transition into Downward Facing Dog (Adho Mukha Svanasana): This pose calms the mind and energizes the body.

4. Close with a brief Breath Awareness exercise: Sit comfortably, close your eyes, and focus on the flow of your breath.

Mindful Yoga Sequence for Evening Relaxation

End your day on a peaceful note with this soothing sequence.

1. Begin in Child's Pose (Balasana): This restful pose is perfect for winding down and turning inward.

2. Move into Legs-Up-The-Wall Pose (Viparita Karani): This gentle inversion calms the nervous system and promotes relaxation.

3. Transition to Reclining Bound Angle Pose (Supta Baddha Konasana): This restorative pose opens the chest and promotes deep, soothing breaths.

4. End with a brief Body Scan Meditation: As you lie in Savasana (Corpse Pose), mentally scan your body from head to toe, releasing tension from each part.

These mindful yoga sequences are not just about the poses, but about the awareness you bring to each pose, each breath, and each moment. They serve as mini-retreats amidst the hustle and bustle of daily life. Remember, every moment you spend on your yoga mat is a step towards greater mindfulness and tranquility. So, breathe deep, stay present, and embrace the beautiful journey of mindful yoga. You, my friend, are on the path to becoming a true mindful maestro!

The Gentle Art of Unwinding: A Deep Dive into Restorative Yoga

Are you prepared to delve into a side of yoga that centers on rejuvenation, tranquility, and gentle release? As we continue our exploration of yoga as a path to relaxation and mindfulness, it's time to spread out the soothing blanket of Restorative Yoga, an enticing invitation to let go and deeply relax.

Understanding Restorative Yoga: More Than Just Relaxation

Restorative Yoga, a unique style that encourages deep relaxation and release, is often described as the antidote to stress. But it's so much more than just a downtime for your body and mind. It's about understanding and appreciating the art of active relaxation.

In Restorative Yoga, the emphasis isn't on stretching or strengthening but rather on releasing tension and sinking into a state of deep relaxation. Unlike traditional yoga, where poses are held for a few breaths, Restorative Yoga encourages you to hold poses for an extended period, often five minutes or even longer.

What sets Restorative Yoga apart is the use of props such as bolsters, blankets, blocks, and yoga straps. These props fully support your body in each pose, allowing your muscles to completely relax and open through passive stretching. Think of these props as your personal assistants, helping you get into and maintain poses with comfort and ease.

The Beauty and Benefits of Restorative Yoga

Restorative Yoga, with its slow pace and focus on relaxation, might seem inactive or easy at first glance. But beneath its serene surface, a profound transformation occurs. It's like the calm, steady process of a caterpillar metamorphosing into a butterfly. Here are some remarkable benefits that this soothing practice offers:

1. Deep Relaxation: The essence of Restorative Yoga is relaxation - deep, wholesome relaxation that permeates every cell in your body. By holding supported poses for longer periods and synchronizing your breath, Restorative Yoga allows you to release deeply held tension and stress. It's like stepping into a warm bath after a long day, where every muscle, every fibre in your body uncoils and unwinds.

2. Stress Relief: Restorative Yoga is a powerful stress buster. The calming, slow-paced nature of the practice signals your body to switch from the 'fight or flight' mode to the 'rest and digest' mode. This triggers the parasympathetic nervous system, your body's natural relaxation response, leading to reduced stress and anxiety levels.

3. Enhanced Flexibility: While there's no active stretching in Restorative Yoga, don't underestimate its power to improve flexibility. The extended hold times in each pose allow your muscles to relax deeply. This gentle release of tension can, over time, lead to increased flexibility and range of motion.

4. Mind-Body Connection: Restorative Yoga provides a beautiful platform to cultivate mindfulness and strengthen the connection between your mind and body. As you settle into a pose and turn your attention inward, you become more attuned to your body's subtle signals, your breath, and the ebb and flow of your thoughts and emotions.

A Glimpse into Restorative Yoga Practice

A typical Restorative Yoga practice would include a series of restful poses that are held for extended periods. Here are a few examples:

1. Supported Child's Pose (Balasana): In this deeply soothing pose, you kneel on the floor, separate your knees about hip-width apart, and extend your torso forward over a bolster or folded blanket that's nestled between your thighs. Your forehead can rest on the bolster, or turn to one side. This pose gently stretches your lower back and hips, releasing tension and promoting a sense of calm and safety.

2. Legs-Up-The-Wall Pose (Viparita Karani): This gentle inversion involves lying on your back with your legs resting against a wall. Your buttocks can be a few inches away from the wall or touching the wall, depending on your comfort. You can place a folded blanket or bolster under your hips to elevate the pelvis. This pose reverses the effects of gravity on your legs and feet, offering relief from fatigue. It also encourages a calming effect on your nervous system.

3. Supported Savasana (Corpse Pose): Arguably the most important pose in any yoga practice, Savasana in a restorative practice often includes multiple props to support the body. Lying on your back, use a bolster or rolled blanket under your knees to relieve tension in the lower back. You can also place a small pillow or folded towel under your head. Close your eyes and allow your body to sink into the mat, releasing tension with every exhale.

Restorative Yoga is like a quiet, peaceful island in the vast, tumultuous ocean of daily life. It offers a haven where you can lay down your burdens, soften your defenses, and allow yourself to simply 'be.' It's a reminder of the importance of rest in our fast-paced world, an invitation to slow down and tune in to our own rhythm.

So, when life gets overwhelming, roll out your yoga mat, gather your props, and surrender to the healing, restorative power of Restorative Yoga. This gentle practice is an ode to relaxation, a celebration of slowing down, and a journey to inner peace. Because you, dear yogi, deserve to rest, to rejuvenate, and to rediscover the joy of simply being. Embrace Restorative Yoga and let its magic heal, restore, and renew you from the inside out!

Inner Harmony: A Guide to Meditation for Mind-Body Healing

As we continue to journey down the path of relaxation and mindfulness, let's explore the potent practice of meditation and its capacity for fostering mind-body healing.

Decoding Meditation: The Path to Wholeness

At its core, meditation is the practice of calming the mind, turning inward, and fostering a deep state of relaxation and alertness. But meditation is more than a method for relaxation. It is a pathway to self-discovery and a tool for fostering harmony between the mind and the body.

Mind-body healing, or the idea that our thoughts, beliefs, and attitudes can affect our physical health, is a cornerstone of many traditional healing practices. In recent decades, this approach has gained attention in the West, with a growing body of research highlighting the role of the mind in health and disease.

Meditation is a vital practice for promoting mind-body healing. Through meditation, we can cultivate a more positive mental state, reduce stress, and promote relaxation - all of which have significant benefits for our physical health.

The Science of Meditation and Mind-Body Healing

Research has shown that regular meditation can bring about changes in our bodies at a physiological level. These changes can lead to a reduction in symptoms of stress-related conditions, enhance our immune response, and promote overall health and well-being. Here are some science-backed benefits of meditation for mind-body healing:

1. Reduces Stress: Meditation has been shown to decrease levels of the stress hormone cortisol. High cortisol levels, associated with chronic stress, can lead to various health problems, including heart disease, sleep problems, and depression.

2. Enhances Immune Function: Regular meditation can boost the function of the immune system, making you more resistant to viruses and infections.

3. Lowers Blood Pressure: Meditation can lead to a reduction in blood pressure, which is beneficial for heart health.

4. Promotes Better Sleep: Regular meditation can help combat insomnia and improve the quality of sleep.

5. Improves Mental Health: Meditation can help decrease symptoms of anxiety and depression, fostering better mental health, which is intrinsically linked to physical well-being.

A Guide to Mind-Body Healing Meditation

Now that we understand the 'why' let's explore the 'how.' Here's a simple meditation practice aimed at fostering mind-body healing:

1. Find a Quiet Place: Choose a quiet, comfortable space where you won't be disturbed. This could be a corner of your room, a spot in your garden, or even a peaceful place in a nearby park.

2. Assume a Comfortable Position: You can sit on a cushion, chair, or even lie down if that's more comfortable for you. The key is to ensure that your body is relaxed and your spine is straight.

3. Close Your Eyes and Relax: Close your eyes and consciously relax your body, releasing tension from each part, starting from the top of your head and moving down to your toes.

4. Focus on Your Breath: Bring your attention to your breath, noticing how your body moves with each inhalation and exhalation. Don't try to control or change your breath, simply observe it.

5. Use a Healing Mantra: Introduce a healing mantra or affirmation. It could be something like, "I am healing," or "Every cell in my body is healthy and strong." Repeat this mantra silently to yourself as you continue to breathe naturally.

6. Practice Regularly: Aim to practice this meditation daily. Consistency is key when it comes to meditation.

Meditation Practice 1: Breath Awareness Meditation

Breath Awareness Meditation is a simple yet powerful practice that focuses on the natural rhythm of your breath.

1. Begin by finding a quiet and comfortable place where you won't be disturbed.

2. Sit comfortably with your spine upright, close your eyes, and relax your body.

3. Bring your attention to your breath, noticing the sensation of the breath entering and leaving your nostrils.

4. As you inhale, mentally note "inhaling," and as you exhale, note "exhaling."

5. If your mind wanders, gently bring your focus back to your breath.

Meditation Practice 2: Loving-Kindness Meditation (Metta Bhavana)

Loving-kindness meditation focuses on cultivating love and kindness towards yourself and others.

1. Find a comfortable and quiet place for meditation. Sit with your back straight and close your eyes.

2. Start by picturing yourself and repeating, "May I be happy. May I be well. May I be safe. May I live with ease."

3. Next, picture someone you love deeply. Repeat the phrases, sending love and positivity their way.

4. Now, visualize someone neutral, perhaps a neighbor or a stranger you saw today. Send them the same loving wishes.

5. Finally, think of someone you have difficulties with. If you feel ready, repeat the same phrases for them.

Meditation Practice 3: Body Scan Meditation

Body Scan Meditation involves paying attention to different parts of your body, from your toes to the crown of your head.

1. Find a comfortable place where you can lie down without being disturbed.

2. Close your eyes and take a few deep breaths to center yourself.

3. Start by bringing your awareness to your toes, then your feet, ankles, and continue to move up your body.

4. At each body part, notice any sensations, tension, or relaxation present without judgment.

5. Continue this scan up through your body until you reach the top of your head.

Meditation Practice 4: Mindfulness Meditation

Mindfulness meditation teaches you to remain aware and present in the moment.

1. Find a quiet, comfortable place to sit with your back straight.

2. Close your eyes and take a few deep breaths, letting your breath return to its natural rhythm.

3. Broaden your awareness to encompass your body and surroundings. Notice sounds, smells, and the sensation of your clothes against your skin.

4. If your mind wanders into thoughts, memories, or plans, gently guide it back to the present moment.

These four meditation practices offer diverse paths to the same destination – a state of inner calm, enhanced awareness, and emotional balance. Remember, there's no 'one-size-fits-all' in meditation. Feel free to explore these practices and find the ones that resonate with you the most.

As we proceed along the path of yoga for relaxation and mindfulness, we now delve into more advanced meditation techniques. These techniques can enhance your meditation practice, providing new dimensions of awareness and inner tranquility.

Meditation Technique 1: Insight Meditation (Vipassana)

Insight Meditation, also known as Vipassana, aims to cultivate a deeper understanding of the nature of reality. It's a practice that focuses on the deep interconnection between mind and body, explored through focused attention to the physical sensations that form the life experience.

1. Begin in a quiet and comfortable place, taking your usual meditation posture.

2. Bring your attention to your breath, observing each inhalation and exhalation.

3. Gradually shift your attention from the breath to the sensations in your body. Notice the feelings associated with each breath - how it affects your chest, your rib cage, your belly.

4. Expand your awareness to include all the physical sensations in your body and any associated thoughts or feelings that arise.

5. Practice non-judgmental observation, acknowledging things as they are without attachment or aversion.

Meditation Technique 2: Zen Meditation (Zazen)

Zen meditation, or Zazen, is the heart of Zen Buddhist practice. The aim of Zazen is to simply sit and suspend all judgmental thinking, letting words, ideas, images, and thoughts pass by without getting involved in them.

1. Sit on a cushion (zafu) in a quiet space, assuming a comfortable posture. You may choose to sit in full or half lotus or kneel. Keep your back straight.

2. Place your hands in the cosmic mudra (right hand supporting the left one, palms up, with thumbs gently touching).

3. Half-close your eyes and direct your gaze downwards, about 3 feet in front of you.

4. Breathe naturally through your nose. Let go of all deliberate thought and let your mind be quiet.

As you dive deeper into the ocean of meditation, these advanced techniques offer you further tools to explore your inner landscape and enrich your meditation journey. They will challenge you, inspire you, and lead you to greater depths of understanding and peace.

Remember, the path of meditation is not always easy. There may be times when these practices seem challenging or even frustrating. But with patience, consistency, and a gentle spirit, you will discover a profound peace and understanding within you, waiting to be unveiled.

So, keep exploring, dear meditator. Embrace the journey with an open heart and a curious mind. You are on a beautiful path of inner discovery, a journey that opens doors to deep peace, heightened awareness, and profound connection with the universe. Enjoy the journey, every step of the way!

Nurturing Mindfulness: The Art of Walking Meditation

Ready to put a refreshing spin on your meditation practice? As we delve deeper into the realm of relaxation and mindfulness through yoga, let's embrace the practice of Walking Meditation - a practice that integrates the tranquility of mindfulness with the natural, soothing rhythm of walking.

Understanding Walking Meditation

Unlike most forms of meditation that require you to sit quietly, Walking Meditation is all about mindful movement. It's a practice where you bring your attention to the physical experience of walking, staying present with each step and the sensation of movement.

The beauty of Walking Meditation is its flexibility. It can be practiced anywhere - in a quiet room, in your backyard, a local park, or during your daily walk. Whether your steps are slow and deliberate or at your normal walking pace, the key is to walk mindfully, with awareness.

The Impact and Benefits of Walking Meditation

Walking Meditation has a broad range of benefits that extend from physical to psychological:

1. Enhances Mindfulness: By focusing on the sensation of walking, you cultivate mindfulness, anchoring yourself in the present moment.

2. Boosts Physical Health: Walking Meditation merges the benefits of physical exercise with meditation. It can help improve cardiovascular health, increase energy levels, and promote better sleep.

3. Relieves Stress: The combination of movement, deep breathing, and mindfulness makes Walking Meditation a potent stress reliever.

4. Connects You with Nature: If practiced outside, Walking Meditation can deepen your connection with nature, enhancing feelings of peace and tranquility.

Walking Meditation: Step-by-Step Guide

Now that we've explored the 'what' and 'why' of Walking Meditation, let's delve into the 'how':

1. Find a Peaceful Place: Choose a quiet and safe place where you can walk undisturbed. An open space with less traffic or a peaceful garden path can be ideal.

2. Begin Walking: Start walking at a comfortable pace. Let it be natural and effortless.

3. Focus on Sensations: Bring your attention to the sensation of your feet making contact with the ground. Feel the weight of your body shifting from one foot to the other.

4. Coordinate with Breath: Try to coordinate your steps with your breath. For example, you might take a step with each inhale and each exhale. Find a rhythm that feels comfortable for you.

5. Practice Mindful Observation: As you walk, broaden your awareness to include the sights, sounds, and smells around you. However, keep your primary focus on the act of walking and the sensation of movement.

6. Gentle Return: If your mind wanders, gently guide your attention back to your walking.

Walking Meditation is a beautiful practice that offers a refreshing way to cultivate mindfulness and tranquility. It's a testament to the fact that meditation doesn't have to be stationary; it can be woven into our everyday movements.

With each mindful step, you're not just moving in space; you're journeying towards inner peace, greater awareness, and holistic well-being.

In the Realm of Resonance: A Deep Dive into Mantra Meditation

Are you ready to experience the transformative power of sound in your meditation journey? As we delve deeper into the enlightening world of yoga for relaxation and mindfulness, we're opening the door to the resonant practice of Mantra Meditation. This practice taps into the vibrational energy of sound, deepening our awareness and inviting tranquility into our lives.

Unfolding Mantra Meditation: A Symphony of Consciousness

Mantra Meditation, also known as Japa Meditation in traditional yogic terms, is a unique form of meditation that utilizes the repetition of a mantra. In Sanskrit, 'mantra' is a compound of two words - 'man,' meaning mind, and 'tra,' meaning tool or instrument. Thus, a mantra is essentially a 'tool of the mind,' a potent sound or vibration that guides our consciousness into quieter, more profound depths.

Mantras in this practice can take various forms. Some people prefer traditional Sanskrit mantras, such as 'Om' or 'Om Shanti,' each carrying a particular vibration and meaning. Others may choose affirmations in their native language that reflect their intentions or goals, such as 'I am calm' or 'I radiate love.' Regardless of its linguistic structure, the mantra serves as a focal point for the mind, a sonic beacon guiding you toward inner peace and clarity.

The Impact and Benefits of Mantra Meditation: Healing through Sound

Mantra Meditation goes beyond the mere act of vocal or mental repetition. It is an immersive practice that harnesses the power of sound vibrations to steer our awareness away from the restless chatter of the mind and into a state of serenity and equilibrium. This shift from sound to silence brings about numerous benefits:

1. Enhances Focus and Concentration: The continual repetition of a mantra anchors the mind, helping to hone concentration skills and improve mental clarity.

2. Induces Relaxation: The rhythmic repetition of a mantra can soothe the nervous system, reducing stress and inducing a deep state of relaxation.

3. Facilitates Mindfulness: By centering your attention on a mantra, you become more attuned to the present moment, fostering a state of mindfulness.

4. Aligns Energy Centers: According to yogic philosophy, specific mantras can help balance the energy centers, or chakras, in the body, promoting overall well-being and a sense of harmony within oneself.

Embarking on the Mantra Meditation Journey: A Detailed Guide

Now that we have a comprehensive understanding of the 'what' and 'why' of Mantra Meditation, let's delve into the 'how'. Here's a detailed guide on how to embark on your Mantra Meditation journey:

1. Selecting Your Mantra: Start by choosing a mantra that resonates with you. This could be a traditional Sanskrit mantra, a word or phrase in your native language, or even a sound that feels soothing and meaningful to you.

2. Creating Your Sacred Space: Find a serene spot that inspires tranquility and is free from disturbances. This space could be in your home, or outdoors amidst nature - wherever you feel at peace.

3. Cultivating Comfort: Position yourself comfortably, ensuring your spine is straight but not tense. You may choose to sit on a meditation cushion on the floor, on a chair, or even against a wall for back support.

4. Beginning the Chant: With your eyes gently closed, begin to repeat your chosen mantra. This repetition can be vocal, whispered, or mental, depending on your comfort level.

5. Focusing on the Sound: As you repeat the mantra, let your attention absorb the sound and rhythm. Try to immerse yourself in the resonance of the mantra, experiencing its vibrational energy.

6. Practicing Non-Judgment: It's natural for the mind to wander or for distractions to arise during meditation. If this happens, gently bring your focus back to the mantra without judging yourself or the distraction.

7. Establishing Regularity: Strive for consistency in your practice, aiming for a set duration each day - 10-20 minutes is often a good starting point.

Mantra Meditation is a dynamic journey of sound, silence, and self-exploration. It's a testament to the power of vibration and the profound impact it can have on our mind and body. As you weave this practice into your daily life, you're not just chanting a series of sounds; you're actively steering your consciousness towards tranquility, balance, and inner harmony.

So, as you continue your exploration of yoga for relaxation and mindfulness, remember that each mantra, each moment spent in meditation, is a step towards a deeper connection with yourself. Embrace the journey, and allow the transformative power of Mantra Meditation to permeate your being, one sound at a time. You are on a glorious path of inner discovery, a path that leads to profound peace, heightened awareness, and resonant harmony. Enjoy each step, each sound, each moment!

Healing Flow: A Yoga Practice for Post-COVID Recovery

Ready to embrace a gentle, restorative yoga practice to aid your post-COVID recovery journey? As we explore yoga's bountiful offerings for relaxation and mindfulness, we're turning our attention to a gentle, nurturing practice, specifically curated to support those recovering from COVID-19.

Before we start, it's crucial to note that each individual's post-COVID recovery will be unique, depending on the severity of the disease and individual health factors. Always listen to your body, move within your comfort zone, and consult with your healthcare provider before starting or modifying any exercise regimen.

Post-COVID recovery can be a challenging time, with individuals experiencing lingering symptoms like fatigue, breathlessness, and anxiety. Yoga, with its emphasis on gentle movement, breathwork, and relaxation, can offer supportive tools to aid in the recovery process:

1. Enhances Lung Capacity: Yoga can help enhance lung capacity and promote efficient breathing, which can be especially beneficial following a respiratory illness like COVID-19.

2. Reduces Stress and Anxiety: The calming and centering effects of yoga can help manage stress and anxiety, often heightened in post-illness recovery periods.

3. Promotes Energy and Strength: Gentle yoga poses can help rebuild strength and energy levels gradually and safely.

This sequence includes gentle asanas (poses) and pranayama (breathing exercises) aimed at improving breath control, reducing anxiety, and enhancing overall well-being.

Remember, take your time with each pose, listen to your body, and modify as needed.

1. Corpse Pose (Savasana): Begin by lying flat on your back on a yoga mat. Allow your body to relax completely, breathing naturally. Stay here for a few minutes, simply focusing on your breath.

2. Seated Deep Breathing: Transition to a comfortable seated position. Rest your hands on your knees and close your eyes. Inhale deeply, filling your lungs with air, then exhale fully, releasing the breath slowly. Repeat this deep, mindful breathing for a few minutes.

3. Cat-Cow Stretch: Move onto your hands and knees in a tabletop position. On an inhale, arch your back, letting your belly drop towards the floor and lift your head and tailbone (Cow pose). On an exhale, round your spine and drop your head and tailbone, pressing the floor away with your hands (Cat pose). Repeat this flow for several breaths, moving at your own pace.

4. Child's Pose (Balasana): From tabletop position, spread your knees wide and sit back on your heels. Stretch your arms in front of you and rest your forehead on the mat. Stay in this pose for a few breaths, feeling a gentle stretch in your back.

5. Seated Twist (Ardha Matsyendrasana): Come to a seated position with your legs extended in front of you. Bend your right knee and place your right foot outside your left thigh. Twist your torso to the right, placing your right hand behind you for support and your left elbow on the outside of your right knee. Hold for a few breaths, then repeat on the other side.

6. Legs-Up-The-Wall Pose (Viparita Karani): Position yourself so your right side is touching a wall. Carefully swing your legs up onto the wall as you pivot to lay on your back. Your body should form a 90-degree angle against the wall. Relax into this pose, allowing gravity to aid in the circulation of blood and lymphatic fluid. Stay in this pose for a few minutes.

7. Final Relaxation (Savasana): End your practice by lying flat on your back in Corpse pose, allowing your body to relax completely. Stay in this pose for several minutes, returning to your natural breath.

This gentle yoga sequence is designed to support your post-COVID recovery, helping you regain strength, flexibility, and breath control at a comfortable pace. As you move through this practice, remember to respect your body's limits and pace yourself.

As you continue on your journey of healing and recovery, let yoga be your ally, aiding in the restoration of balance, vitality, and well-being. You are a picture of resilience and strength, and every mindful movement and breath brings you one step closer to health and vitality. You've got this!

The Healing Embrace of Sleep: The Pivotal Role of Restful Slumber in Post-COVID Recovery

It's time to turn our attention to another critical, albeit frequently underestimated aspect of wellness - sleep. A rejuvenating night's sleep plays a vital role in healing and recovery, making it a cornerstone of your journey back to health.

Why Sleep Matters in Post-COVID Recovery

The restorative power of sleep goes far beyond simple rest. During sleep, our bodies enter a state of deep restoration, facilitating crucial healing processes. This becomes particularly important when your body is recovering from an illness such as COVID-19.

1. *Restoration and Healing:* During the deeper stages of sleep, our bodies release growth hormones that play a vital role in cell repair and regeneration. This natural restorative process supports physical recovery from illness and injury.

2. *Boosting Immune Function:* Adequate, quality sleep is essential for a robust immune system. During sleep, our bodies produce and deploy cytokines, proteins that play a critical role in modulating our immune response and inflammation.

3. *Mental Health and Emotional Well-being:* Good sleep is also a cornerstone of mental health. It helps regulate mood, reduce stress, and alleviate anxiety levels, which can be heightened during a recovery period.

Strategies for Cultivating Restful Sleep During Recovery

Sleep disturbances can be common during the recovery process, but there are strategies that can help improve your sleep quality:

1. *Establish a Consistent Sleep Schedule:* Regular sleep and wake times can help regulate your body's internal clock, or circadian rhythm, improving your sleep quality.

2. *Optimize Daytime Naps:* Rest during recovery is essential, but try to limit daytime naps to 30 minutes or less to avoid disrupting your nighttime sleep.

3. *Create a Serene Sleep Environment:* Aim for a sleep environment that is cool, dark, and quiet. Consider using earplugs, a white noise machine, or a sleep mask to block out disturbances.

4. *Develop a Pre-Sleep Ritual:* Create a calming bedtime routine that signals to your body that it's time for sleep. This could include practices like reading, taking a warm bath, gentle yoga stretches, or meditation.

5. *Be Mindful of Your Diet:* Aim to limit caffeine intake, especially in the latter part of the day, and avoid large meals close to bedtime. Stay well-hydrated during the day, but taper off your fluid intake in the evening to minimize nighttime bathroom trips.

6. *Integrate Bedtime Yoga and Meditation:* Gentle yoga sequences designed for sleep preparation or guided sleep meditations can create a state of relaxation, preparing your mind and body for restful sleep.

Remember, restful sleep is not a luxury but a fundamental necessity for your recovery. It is just as critical as your nutrition, hydration, and your yoga, pranayama, and meditation practices. As you navigate your recovery journey, strive to achieve a balanced harmony among these vital elements of wellness.

Every deep breath, every mindful movement, every nourishing meal, and every restful night's sleep marks a step towards your recovery and vibrant health. You embody resilience, and every day on this healing journey is a testament to your inner strength and fortitude.

Embrace this journey with an open heart and a patient spirit. Grant yourself the kindness and grace to recover at your body's natural pace. Your path is one of restoration and rejuvenation, and with each day, you grow stronger and healthier. Keep going, valiant soul, you're on your way to reclaiming your vibrant wellness! Here's to your unwavering spirit and tenacious resilience. You're doing a fantastic job!

Pathway to Restoration: An In-Depth 30-Day Yoga, Pranayama, and Meditation Regimen for Post-COVID Recovery

Are you ready to venture on a healing journey towards wellness, harnessing the nurturing power of yoga, pranayama, and meditation? As we deepen our exploration of yoga for relaxation and mindfulness, we're presenting a detailed 30-day program, meticulously designed to aid your recovery from COVID-19. This gentle, restorative regimen focuses on enhancing lung capacity, rebuilding strength, and fostering emotional healing.

Before embarking on this journey, ensure to consult your healthcare provider. Be mindful of your body's signals and make modifications as necessary. The primary goal is to gently stimulate recovery, not exert undue strain on your body.

Week 1: Laying the Foundation

Days 1-7: The initial week involves simple breathing exercises and gentle yoga stretches. The objective is to familiarize yourself with yogic practices and start working on lung capacity.

1. *Seated Deep Breathing (5-10 minutes):* Sit comfortably, ensuring your back is straight but not strained. Practice slow, deep inhalations and exhalations. Focus on filling your lungs entirely on each inhale and emptying them completely on each exhale. This pranayama practice will serve as the cornerstone of your 30-day journey.

2. *Gentle Yoga (15-20 minutes):* Start with basic poses such as the Cat-Cow Stretch for spine flexibility, Child's Pose for a gentle back stretch, and Seated Forward Bend for hamstring flexibility. Remember to move into and out of each pose with your breath, synchronizing your movements with your inhales and exhales.

3. *Mindfulness Meditation (5-10 minutes):* Close your day with a short mindfulness meditation. Sit comfortably, close your eyes, and focus on your breath. Observe the sensation of the breath moving in and out of your nostrils and the rise and fall of your abdomen as you breathe.

Week 2: Cultivating Strength

Days 8-14: As you become more attuned to the practices, introduce more strength-building asanas.

1. *Seated Deep Breathing (5-10 minutes)*

2. *Yoga (20-30 minutes):* Continue practicing the poses from Week 1 and gradually introduce strength-building poses. Mountain Pose for posture alignment, Warrior II for lower body strength, and Tree Pose for balance and focus can be included.

3. *Mindfulness Meditation (10 minutes):* Try a guided body scan meditation. This practice helps cultivate body awareness and promotes relaxation. Start at one end of your body (the top of your head or the tips of your toes) and slowly move your attention through your entire body, observing any sensations you feel along the way.

Week 3: Expanding Breath Capacity

Days 15-21: This week introduces simple pranayama exercises to improve lung capacity further.

1. *Seated Deep Breathing (5-10 minutes)*

2. *Pranayama (10-15 minutes):* Begin practicing Full Yogic Breath, a deep breathing technique that engages all three sections of the lungs. Start by filling the lower part of your lungs (belly), then the middle part (lower chest), and finally the upper part (upper chest and throat). Exhale smoothly in the reverse order.

3. *Yoga (20-30 minutes):* Introduce poses like Bridge Pose for gentle backbend and chest opening, and Sphinx Pose for upper body stretch and stress relief.

4. *Meditation (10 minutes):* Continue with the body scan meditation or try a loving-kindness meditation. This form of meditation focuses on developing feelings of goodwill, kindness, and warmth towards oneself and others, fostering emotional healing.

Week 4: Deepening the Practice

Days 22-30: Now that your body is more familiar with the practices, focus on more prolonged yoga sessions and in-depth breathwork.

1. *Pranayama (10-15 minutes):* Continue with Full Yogic Breath and introduce Alternate Nostril Breathing (Nadi Shodhana). This pranayama technique helps balance the body's energy channels and calm the mind.

2. *Yoga (30-40 minutes):* Gradually incorporate poses like Cobra Pose for chest opening and strengthening the back, Downward Dog for overall body stretch, and Legs-Up-The-Wall pose for relaxation. Always end your session with Savasana (Corpse Pose), allowing your body a few minutes to absorb the benefits of your practice.

3. *Meditation (10-15 minutes):* Gradually extend your meditation time. You can continue focusing on your breath or try mantra meditation, repeating a word or phrase that has a positive meaning for you.

This comprehensive 30-day program provides a structured pathway to harness yoga, pranayama, and meditation's healing potential in your post-COVID recovery. Remember, the essence of this journey lies in patience, gentle progression, and honoring your body's needs.

As you step onto this path of restoration, understand that progress may be gradual, and that's perfectly alright. Each day, each practice signifies your resilience, strength, and commitment towards recovery. Each moment you spend on the mat is a moment spent in self-care, a step closer to vibrant health and wellness. Keep going, brave soul! Embrace this journey with open arms and a hopeful heart, for you are on your way to rejuvenation and vitality. Here's to your health and resilience!